System Upgrade:

Reprogramming Metabolism After 50

By: Zafar Khan

Table of Contents

About The Author

Zafar Khan is a seasoned professional with a strong academic background, holding a Master of Science in Statistics and a Master's degree in Computer Science. With over two decades of experience in the Middle East, he has worked with several prestigious multinational companies, including GlaxoSmithKline, Siemens, Cisco, and Nokia.

In August 2023, Zafar was diagnosed with Metabolic Syndrome and Type 2 Diabetes, which sparked a profound interest in healthcare. This personal journey has led him to dedicate his time to learning about self-care, prevention, and functional medicine, with the aim of extending life span and health span for himself and others.

Zafar is actively engaged in educating the public about these topics through various platforms. He maintains a robust social media presence, where he shares insights and resources related to health and wellness. You can find him on his website at www.WulfWorld.com, as well as on YouTube, Instagram, and TikTok under the handle @UnlockMetabolicHealth.

Part I: My Journey to Metabolic Health

Chapter 1: Sharing the Journey

1.1 Becoming an Advocate for Metabolic Health

My journey with metabolic syndrome and type 2 diabetes began with a grim diagnosis and a daunting prognosis. Like many, I was faced with the conventional medical approach: a lifelong dependence on medication to manage my blood sugar levels. However, I chose a different path—a path of complete lifestyle transformation. Through diligent changes in diet, exercise, sleep, and stress management, I successfully reversed my condition. This personal victory ignited a passion within me to help others realize that they too can reclaim their health.

Becoming an advocate for metabolic health was a natural progression from my personal journey. I understood the fear, frustration, and helplessness that accompany a diagnosis of metabolic syndrome or type 2 diabetes. I also knew the empowerment that comes with taking control of one's health. My advocacy started with sharing my story—openly and honestly—about the struggles, setbacks, and triumphs along the way. I wanted to be a beacon of hope for others, showing them that reversing these conditions is possible without resorting to drugs.

1.2 Tips for Supporting Others on Their Journey

Supporting others on their journey to better metabolic health requires empathy, knowledge, and practical strategies. Here are some tips that I have found effective:

1.2.1 Listen and Understand

Every individual's experience with metabolic syndrome and type 2 diabetes is unique. Listening to their stories and understanding their challenges is the first step in providing meaningful support.

1.2.2 Education is Key

Many people are unaware of how lifestyle changes can significantly impact their health. Educating them about the importance of diet, exercise, sleep, and stress management is crucial. Share credible resources, personal anecdotes, and scientific evidence to reinforce your points.

1.2.3 Set Realistic Goals

Encourage setting small, achievable goals rather than overwhelming them with drastic changes. This could be as simple as incorporating more vegetables into their diet, walking for 30 minutes a day, or establishing a regular sleep routine.

1.2.4 Be a Role Model

Lead by example. When others see the positive changes in your health and lifestyle, they are more likely to be inspired to follow suit. Demonstrate healthy eating habits, regular exercise routines, and effective stress management techniques.

1.2.5 Provide Emotional Support

The journey to reversing metabolic syndrome and type 2 diabetes can be emotionally taxing. Offer a shoulder to lean on, celebrate their successes, and provide encouragement during setbacks.

1.2.6 Create a Supportive Community

Encourage them to join support groups or online communities where they can connect with others who are on similar journeys. Sharing experiences and tips can be incredibly motivating and reassuring.

1.2.7 Customize Advice

Recognize that what worked for you may not work for everyone. Customize your advice based on their preferences, lifestyle, and health conditions. Flexibility and personalization are key to sustainable changes.

1.3 The Bigger Picture: Changing the Diabetes Paradigm

As we share our stories and support others on their journey, we contribute to a larger movement—changing the diabetes paradigm. The conventional approach to managing type 2 diabetes often focuses on medication and managing symptoms rather than addressing the root causes. By advocating for lifestyle changes, we challenge this paradigm and promote a more holistic, sustainable approach to health.

This shift requires a collective effort. Healthcare providers, policymakers, and communities need to recognize the power of lifestyle interventions. Integrating nutrition education, physical activity programs, stress management workshops, and sleep hygiene into public health strategies can create a supportive environment for individuals to thrive.

Moreover, it is essential to address the socio-economic factors that contribute to the prevalence of metabolic syndrome and type 2 diabetes. Access to healthy food, safe spaces for physical activity, and affordable healthcare are critical components of a supportive environment. Advocacy efforts should also focus on these broader issues to create lasting change.

In conclusion, my journey from a diagnosis of metabolic syndrome and type 2 diabetes to becoming an advocate for metabolic health has been transformative. By sharing my story, supporting others, and challenging the conventional approach to diabetes management, I aim to contribute to a healthier, more empowered society. Together, we can change the narrative and help countless individuals reclaim their health and lives.

Chapter 2: My Diagnosis and Wake-up Call

2.1 The Day Everything Changed

August 2023 marked a pivotal moment in my life, one that I never saw coming. At 51 years old, I had always prided myself on maintaining what I believed to be a healthy lifestyle. I exercised regularly, made conscious dietary choices, and steered clear of harmful habits like smoking and excessive alcohol consumption. In my mind, I was doing everything right to ensure a long and healthy life.

However, life had a different plan for me. On that fateful day in August, I sat in my doctor's office, anxiously awaiting the results of my recent health check-up. The words that followed would change the course of my life forever: "You have Metabolic Syndrome and Type II Diabetes."

The diagnosis hit me like a ton of bricks. How could this be possible? I had always considered myself to be in good health. The shock was palpable, and for a moment, I felt as if the ground beneath me had shifted. This wasn't just a minor health hiccup; it was a serious condition that required immediate attention and action.

As my doctor explained the implications of the diagnosis, I found myself struggling to process the information. Metabolic Syndrome, a cluster of conditions that increase the risk of heart disease, stroke, and diabetes, coupled with Type II Diabetes, a chronic condition affecting the way my body metabolized sugar – it all seemed surreal.

The reality of my situation slowly began to sink in. This diagnosis wasn't just a wake-up call; it was a blaring alarm that demanded immediate action. I realized that despite my perceived healthy lifestyle, there were clearly aspects of my health that I had overlooked or misunderstood.

2.2 Coming to Terms with My Condition

The days following my diagnosis were a whirlwind of emotions. Disbelief, anger, fear, and confusion all vied for dominance in my mind. How could I have developed these conditions despite my best efforts to lead a healthy life? It was a humbling experience that forced me to reevaluate everything I thought I knew about health and wellness.

As I began to research Metabolic Syndrome and Type II Diabetes, I realized that there was so much more to learn about these conditions. I discovered that genetics, age, and even stress levels could play significant roles in their development. It wasn't just about diet and exercise; it was about understanding the complex interplay of various factors affecting my body.

Coming to terms with my condition meant acknowledging that I had been operating under some misconceptions about health. What I had believed to be a healthy lifestyle wasn't necessarily optimal for my individual needs. This realization was both frightening and liberating. On one hand, it meant admitting that I had been wrong about some aspects of my health. On the other hand, it opened up new possibilities for improvement and change.

I also had to confront the potential long-term implications of my diagnosis. Left unchecked, Metabolic Syndrome and Type II Diabetes could lead to serious complications, including heart disease, kidney damage, and vision problems. The gravity of the situation became increasingly clear, and with it came a sense of urgency to take action.

During this period of coming to terms with my condition, I experienced a range of emotions. There were moments of despair when the task ahead seemed insurmountable. But there were also moments of hope, fueled by stories of individuals who had successfully managed and even reversed their conditions through lifestyle changes.

2.3 Deciding to Take Control

As the initial shock of my diagnosis began to subside, a new emotion emerged: determination. I realized that while I couldn't change the fact that I had been diagnosed with Metabolic Syndrome and Type II Diabetes, I could certainly control how I responded to it. This was the moment I decided to take matters into my own hands.

When my doctor presented me with treatment options, including medication, I made a bold decision. I chose to decline medication and instead focus on lifestyle changes to manage my condition. This wasn't a decision I made lightly, but one born out of a deep-seated belief that I could make significant improvements through natural means.

My research had shown me that diet played a crucial role in managing both Metabolic Syndrome and Type II

Diabetes. I decided to adopt a Low Carb, High Fat (LCHF) diet, a nutritional approach that had shown promising results for many individuals with similar conditions. This meant overhauling my entire approach to eating, but I was ready for the challenge.

Exercise, which had always been a part of my routine, now took on new importance. I committed to a more structured and consistent exercise regimen, understanding its vital role in managing blood sugar levels and improving overall metabolic health.

Recognizing the impact of stress and poor sleep on metabolic health, I also decided to establish a strict sleep protocol and implement stress management techniques. This holistic approach felt right to me – addressing not just the physical aspects of my condition, but the mental and emotional components as well.

Taking control meant educating myself, making informed decisions, and being proactive about my health. It meant viewing my diagnosis not as a life sentence, but as an opportunity for positive change. I was no longer a passive recipient of health advice; I was an active participant in my own healing journey.

This decision to take control marked the beginning of a new chapter in my life. It was a commitment to myself, a promise to do whatever it took to improve my health and potentially reverse my condition. The road ahead would be challenging, but I was ready to face it head-on.

As I embarked on this new journey, I felt a mix of anticipation and apprehension. There were many unknowns ahead, but one thing was certain: my life had changed irrevocably on that day in August 2023, and it was up to me to ensure it changed for the better.

Chapter 3: Researching and Planning My Approach

3.1 Diving into the Science

After receiving my diagnosis of metabolic syndrome and type 2 diabetes, I knew I needed to take immediate action. The first step in my journey was to immerse myself in the scientific literature surrounding these conditions. I wanted to understand not just the symptoms and conventional treatments, but also the underlying mechanisms and potential alternative approaches.

My research began with a deep dive into the pathophysiology of metabolic syndrome and type 2 diabetes. I learned about insulin resistance, the role of inflammation, and how these factors contribute to the development and progression of these conditions. This knowledge was crucial in helping me understand why traditional approaches might not be sufficient for everyone.

I explored numerous scientific journals, medical publications, and reputable health websites. The wealth of information was overwhelming at first, but I gradually began to piece together a comprehensive picture of my condition. I paid particular attention to studies on lifestyle interventions, as I was determined to find natural ways to improve my health.

One area that particularly caught my attention was the emerging research on low-carbohydrate, high-fat (LCHF) diets and their potential benefits for metabolic health. I discovered studies suggesting that reducing carbohydrate intake could lead to improved insulin sensitivity and better blood sugar control. This led me to investigate the carnivore diet as well, which some proponents claim can have profound effects on metabolic health.

Exercise was another key area of my research. I delved into studies on different types of physical activity and their impacts on metabolic health. I learned about the benefits of cardio, the concept of Zone 2 training for metabolic flexibility, and the importance of strength and resistance training for improving insulin sensitivity and overall metabolic health.

The science of sleep and its connection to metabolic health was a revelation to me. I studied the intricate relationship between our circadian rhythms and hormone regulation, particularly how disrupted sleep patterns can negatively impact insulin sensitivity and glucose metabolism.

Lastly, I explored the growing body of research on stress management and its effects on metabolic health. I was fascinated by studies showing how chronic stress can contribute to insulin resistance and how mindfulness practices could potentially mitigate these effects.

3.2 Consulting Experts and Finding Support

While my personal research provided a strong foundation, I recognized the importance of seeking professional guidance. I began by consulting with my primary care physician, who provided valuable insights into my condition and helped me interpret my lab results.

Next, I sought out an endocrinologist who specialized in metabolic disorders. This expert was instrumental in helping me understand the nuances of my condition and discussing potential treatment options. They also helped me set realistic goals and expectations for my health journey.

Recognizing the crucial role of nutrition in managing my condition, I scheduled appointments with several registered dietitians. These professionals helped me navigate the complex world of nutrition science and provided practical advice on implementing dietary changes. They were particularly helpful in discussing the pros and cons of LCHF and carnivore diets, ensuring I could make an informed decision about my nutritional approach.

To address the exercise component of my strategy, I consulted with a certified personal trainer who had experience working with individuals with metabolic disorders. They helped me design a balanced exercise program that incorporated cardio, Zone 2 training, strength and resistance exercises, and mobility work.

For guidance on improving my sleep habits, I spoke with a sleep specialist. They provided invaluable advice on optimizing my sleep environment and establishing a consistent sleep schedule to support my circadian rhythm.

To address stress management, I sought out a mental health professional who specialized in mindfulness-based stress reduction techniques. Their guidance was crucial in helping me develop effective strategies for managing stress and its impact on my metabolic health.

Throughout this process, I also connected with support groups and online communities of individuals facing similar health challenges. These connections provided emotional support, practical tips, and a sense of camaraderie that proved invaluable on my journey.

3.3 Developing My Personal Strategy

Armed with scientific knowledge and expert guidance, I set out to develop a comprehensive, personalized strategy to address my metabolic syndrome and type 2 diabetes. I recognized that a multi-faceted approach would be necessary to tackle these complex conditions effectively.

My strategy centered around four key components:

3.3.1 Diet and Nutrition

Based on my research and consultations, I decided to adopt a low-carbohydrate, high-fat (LCHF) approach, with elements of the carnivore diet. This involved drastically reducing my intake of processed carbohydrates and focusing on whole, nutrient-dense foods. I planned my meals to include high-quality proteins, healthy fats, and low-carb vegetables. I also implemented intermittent fasting, which some studies suggested could improve insulin sensitivity.

3.3.2 Exercise

My exercise plan was diverse and comprehensive, designed to address various aspects of metabolic health:
- Cardio: Regular aerobic exercises to improve cardiovascular health and insulin sensitivity.
- Zone 2 Training: Incorporating low-intensity, steady-state exercises to enhance metabolic flexibility.
- Strength and Resistance Training: Weight lifting and bodyweight exercises to build muscle mass and improve glucose metabolism.

- Mobility and Flexibility: Daily stretching and mobility work to support overall physical health and reduce the risk of injuries.

3.3.3 Sleep Optimization

I developed a strict sleep routine to support my circadian rhythm:
- Consistent sleep and wake times, even on weekends.
- Creating a dark, cool, and quiet sleep environment.
- Limiting blue light exposure in the evenings.
- Establishing a relaxing pre-bed routine to signal to my body that it's time to wind down.

3.3.4 Stress Management

To address the impact of stress on my metabolic health, I incorporated several mindfulness practices:
- Daily meditation sessions.
- Regular yoga practice.
- Breathing exercises throughout the day.
- Journaling to process emotions and track my progress.

In addition to these core components, I also planned for regular check-ins with my healthcare providers to monitor my progress and make adjustments as needed. I set up a system to track various health metrics, including blood glucose levels, weight, and subjective measures of well-being.

I recognized that this strategy would require significant lifestyle changes, and I prepared myself mentally for the challenges ahead. I viewed this not as a temporary fix, but as a long-term commitment to my health and well-being.

As I finalized my personal strategy, I felt a sense of empowerment and hope. While the road ahead would undoubtedly be challenging, I was confident that with the knowledge I had gained, the support system I had built, and the comprehensive plan I had developed, I was well-equipped to take control of my health and work towards reversing my metabolic syndrome and type 2 diabetes.

This marked the beginning of a new chapter in my life – one where I would be an active participant in my health journey, armed with science, supported by experts, and guided by a carefully crafted personal strategy.

Chapter 4: Implementing Lifestyle Changes

Metabolic syndrome and type 2 diabetes are increasingly common health challenges that can significantly impact quality of life. However, with the right approach, these conditions can often be managed and even reversed through comprehensive lifestyle changes. This chapter explores the journey of implementing these changes, focusing on diet, exercise, stress management, and sleep optimization.

4.1 Overhauling My Diet

The cornerstone of my strategy to address metabolic syndrome and type 2 diabetes was a complete overhaul of my diet. After extensive research and consultation with healthcare professionals, I decided to adopt a low-carbohydrate, high-fat (LCHF) approach, with elements of the carnivore diet.

4.1.1 LCHF Diet

The LCHF diet involves drastically reducing carbohydrate intake while increasing the consumption of healthy fats. This approach aims to shift the body's primary fuel source from glucose to fat, a state known as nutritional ketosis. Here's how I implemented this change:

1. Carbohydrate Reduction: I gradually reduced my carbohydrate intake to less than 50 grams per day. This meant eliminating sugar, grains, and starchy vegetables from my diet.
2. Increasing Healthy Fats: I incorporated more healthy fats into my meals, including avocados, olive oil, coconut oil, and fatty fish rich in omega-3s.

3. Moderate Protein Intake: I ensured adequate protein intake from sources like eggs, fish, poultry, and lean meats.
4. Non-Starchy Vegetables: I increased my intake of low-carb vegetables like leafy greens, broccoli, and cauliflower to ensure adequate fiber and micronutrient intake.

4.1.2 Carnivore Diet Elements

While not adopting a strict carnivore diet, I incorporated some of its principles:

1. Emphasis on Animal Products: I made animal products the centerpiece of many meals, focusing on grass-fed beef, organ meats, and wild-caught fish.
2. Elimination of Plant Foods: For a period, I experimented with eliminating most plant foods to observe how my body responded.
3. Zero-Carb Days: I occasionally implemented zero-carb days, consuming only animal products.

The results of this dietary shift were significant. Within weeks, I noticed improved blood glucose control, reduced inflammation, and increased energy levels. However, it's important to note that such dramatic dietary changes should always be undertaken under medical supervision, especially for individuals with diabetes or other health conditions.

4.2 Incorporating Exercise

Exercise plays a crucial role in managing metabolic syndrome and type 2 diabetes. I developed a comprehensive exercise regimen that included cardio, strength training, and flexibility work.

4.2.1 Cardio and Zone 2 Training

1. Zone 2 Training: I incorporated regular Zone 2 cardio sessions, typically 3-4 times per week for 45-60 minutes. This involved maintaining a heart rate at about 60-70% of my maximum, which helps improve insulin sensitivity and fat metabolism.
2. High-Intensity Interval Training (HIIT): Once a week, I included a HIIT session to boost cardiovascular fitness and glucose uptake by muscles.

4.2.2 Strength and Resistance Training

1. Full-Body Workouts: I performed full-body strength training workouts 2-3 times per week, focusing on compound movements like squats, deadlifts, bench presses, and rows.
2. Progressive Overload: I gradually increased the weight and complexity of exercises to continually challenge my muscles and improve insulin sensitivity.

4.2.3 Mobility and Flexibility

1. Daily Stretching: I incorporated a 15-minute stretching routine into my daily schedule to improve flexibility and reduce the risk of injury.

2. Yoga: Twice a week, I attended yoga classes to enhance both mobility and mindfulness.

The combination of these exercise modalities not only improved my physical fitness but also had a profound impact on my metabolic health. Regular blood tests showed improvements in insulin sensitivity and lipid profiles.

4.3 Managing Stress and Sleep

Stress management and adequate sleep are often overlooked aspects of metabolic health. I focused on optimizing both to support my overall health goals.

4.3.1 Stress Management

1. Mindfulness Meditation: I began practicing mindfulness meditation for 15-20 minutes daily, using apps like Headspace and Calm for guidance.
2. Deep Breathing Exercises: I incorporated deep breathing exercises throughout the day, especially during stressful moments.
3. Nature Therapy: I made it a point to spend time in nature regularly, whether through hiking, gardening, or simply sitting in a park.
4. Journaling: Daily journaling helped me process emotions and identify stress triggers.

4.3.2 Sleep Optimization

1. Consistent Sleep Schedule: I established a consistent sleep schedule, aiming to sleep and

wake at the same times every day, even on weekends.

2. Sleep Environment: I optimized my bedroom for sleep by ensuring darkness, coolness, and quiet.

3. Digital Sunset: I implemented a "digital sunset" 2 hours before bedtime, avoiding blue light from screens.

4. Bedtime Routine: I developed a relaxing bedtime routine including reading, light stretching, and herbal tea.

These practices significantly reduced my stress levels and improved my sleep quality. As a result, I noticed better glucose control, reduced cravings, and improved overall well-being.

4.4 The Challenges and Triumphs Along the Way

Implementing such comprehensive lifestyle changes was not without its challenges. Here are some of the obstacles I faced and how I overcame them:

4.4.1 Challenges

1. Social Situations: Adhering to a strict LCHF diet in social settings was initially challenging. I learned to plan ahead, communicate my needs, and find LCHF-friendly options in most restaurants.

2. Exercise Consistency: Maintaining a consistent exercise routine amidst a busy schedule was difficult. I overcame this by scheduling workouts like

any other important appointment and finding an accountability partner.
3. Stress Management: Initially, I found it hard to make time for stress management practices. I addressed this by starting small, with just 5 minutes of meditation daily, and gradually increasing the duration.
4. Sleep Discipline: Breaking old habits like late-night TV watching was tough. I used habit stacking techniques, linking my new sleep routine to existing habits to make it stick.

4.4.2 Triumphs

1. Weight Loss: Over six months, I lost 30 pounds, primarily from fat mass.

2. Improved Blood Glucose: My HbA1c dropped from 7.2% to 5.6%, moving me out of the diabetic range.
3. Increased Energy: I experienced a significant boost in energy levels, no longer suffering from the afternoon slumps.
4. Better Sleep: My sleep quality improved dramatically, with fewer wake-ups and more restful nights.
5. Improved Mental Clarity: I noticed enhanced cognitive function and emotional stability.

The journey of implementing these lifestyle changes was transformative. It required dedication, patience, and a willingness to learn and adapt. While the path wasn't always easy, the improvements in my health and quality of life made every challenge worthwhile.

Remember, everyone's journey is unique, and what worked for me may need to be adjusted for others. It's crucial to work with healthcare professionals when making significant lifestyle changes, especially when managing conditions like metabolic syndrome and type 2 diabetes

Part II: Understanding Metabolic Health and Type 2 Diabetes

Chapter 5: The Basics of Metabolism

Metabolism is a term we often hear in discussions about health, weight, and energy. But what exactly does it mean, and why is it so crucial to our overall well-being? In this chapter, we'll dive into the fundamentals of metabolism, explore its key components, and understand how it can sometimes go awry.

5.1 What is Metabolism?

At its core, metabolism refers to all the chemical processes that occur within a living organism to maintain life. These processes involve two main categories:

5.1.1 Catabolism

The breakdown of complex molecules into simpler ones, often releasing energy.

5.1.2 Anabolism

The building of complex molecules from simpler ones, usually requiring energy.

Think of your body as a complex machine. Just as a car needs fuel to run and performs various functions to move forward, your body needs energy to perform all its tasks - from breathing and circulating blood to growing and repairing cells.

Metabolism isn't just about digesting food and burning calories. It encompasses a vast array of processes, including:

- Converting food into energy
- Eliminating waste products
- Regulating body temperature
- Contracting muscles
- Transmitting nerve signals
- And much more

Your metabolic rate - the speed at which your body performs these processes - can vary based on several factors:

1. Age: Metabolism typically slows as we get older.
2. Body composition: Muscle burns more calories than fat, even at rest.
3. Gender: Men often have a faster metabolism than women due to higher muscle mass.
4. Genetics: Some people are born with faster or slower metabolisms.
5. Physical activity: Regular exercise can boost metabolism.
6. Hormones: Various hormones play crucial roles in regulating metabolism.

Understanding your metabolism is the first step towards optimizing your health. It's not just about how quickly you burn calories, but how efficiently your body performs all its necessary functions.

5.2 Key Players: Insulin, Glucose, and Fat

While metabolism involves numerous substances and processes, three key players stand out in discussions of metabolic health: insulin, glucose, and fat. Understanding their roles and interactions is crucial to grasping how metabolism affects our health.

5.2.1 Glucose: The Body's Primary Fuel

Glucose is a simple sugar that serves as the primary energy source for most of our body's cells. When we consume carbohydrates, our digestive system breaks them down into glucose, which enters our bloodstream.

5.2.2 Insulin: The Master Regulator

Insulin is a hormone produced by the pancreas that plays a crucial role in glucose metabolism. Its main functions include:

1. Facilitating glucose uptake: Insulin signals cells to absorb glucose from the bloodstream.
2. Promoting storage: It encourages the liver and muscles to store excess glucose as glycogen.
3. Inhibiting glucose production: Insulin tells the liver to stop producing glucose when blood sugar levels are sufficient.
4. Regulating fat metabolism: It promotes fat storage and inhibits fat breakdown.

5.2.3 Fat: Energy Reserve and Metabolic Player

While often vilified, fat plays essential roles in our metabolism:

1. Energy storage: Fat cells store excess energy for future use.
2. Hormone production: Adipose tissue produces hormones that influence metabolism.
3. Insulation: Body fat helps maintain body temperature.
4. Protection: Fat cushions and protects vital organs.

5.2.4 The Interplay

The interaction between these key players is complex and delicate. After a meal, blood glucose levels rise, triggering insulin release. Insulin then facilitates glucose uptake by cells and storage as glycogen or fat. Between meals, when glucose levels drop, the body begins to break down stored glycogen and fat for energy.

This delicate balance can be disrupted by various factors, leading to metabolic disorders like diabetes.

5.3 When Metabolism Goes Awry

Despite its complexity and built-in regulatory mechanisms, metabolism can sometimes malfunction. These disruptions can lead to various metabolic disorders, with significant impacts on health and quality of life.

5.3.1 Insulin Resistance and Type 2 Diabetes

One of the most common metabolic disorders is insulin resistance, which can lead to type 2 diabetes. In this condition:

1. Cells become less responsive to insulin's signals.
2. The pancreas produces more insulin to compensate.
3. Eventually, the pancreas may struggle to produce enough insulin.
4. Blood glucose levels remain consistently high.

2.3.2 Metabolic Syndrome

Metabolic syndrome is a cluster of conditions that often occur together, increasing the risk of heart disease, stroke, and type 2 diabetes. It includes:

- High blood pressure
- High blood sugar
- Excess body fat around the waist
- Abnormal cholesterol or triglyceride levels

5.3.3 Obesity

While often discussed in terms of weight, obesity is fundamentally a metabolic disorder. It involves:

- Excessive accumulation of body fat
- Hormonal imbalances
- Chronic low-grade inflammation

- Increased risk of other metabolic disorders

5.3.4 Thyroid Disorders

The thyroid gland produces hormones that regulate metabolism. Disorders can lead to:

- Hyperthyroidism: Overactive metabolism
- Hypothyroidism: Underactive metabolism

Both conditions can significantly impact overall health and well-being.

5.3.5 Mitochondrial Disorders

Mitochondria are the "powerhouses" of our cells, responsible for producing energy. Disorders affecting mitochondrial function can have widespread impacts on metabolism and health.

Understanding these metabolic disruptions is crucial for maintaining health and addressing potential issues early. In the following chapters, we'll explore how lifestyle factors can influence these processes and how we can optimize our metabolism for better health.

Chapter 6: Type 2 Diabetes Demystified

Type 2 diabetes is often described as a modern epidemic, affecting millions of people worldwide. Despite its prevalence, there's still much confusion about its causes, risk factors, and long-term effects. In this chapter, we'll demystify type 2 diabetes, providing a clear understanding of this complex metabolic disorder.

6.1 What Causes Type 2 Diabetes?

At its core, type 2 diabetes is a disorder of blood sugar regulation. To understand its causes, we need to delve into the intricate dance between glucose and insulin in our bodies.

6.1.1 The Glucose-Insulin Relationship

In a healthy metabolism:
1. We consume food, which is broken down into glucose.
2. Blood glucose levels rise.
3. The pancreas releases insulin.
4. Insulin helps cells absorb glucose from the blood.
5. Blood glucose levels return to normal.

In type 2 diabetes, this process goes awry:

6.1.2 Insulin Resistance

The primary cause of type 2 diabetes is insulin resistance. This means:
- Cells become less responsive to insulin's signals.

- More insulin is needed to achieve the same blood sugar-lowering effect.
- The pancreas produces more insulin to compensate.
- Over time, the pancreas may struggle to produce enough insulin.

6.1.3 Factors Contributing to Insulin Resistance

Several factors can contribute to the development of insulin resistance:

1. Excess Body Fat: Particularly visceral fat (around organs) can release hormones that interfere with insulin's action.
2. Lack of Physical Activity: Regular exercise helps maintain insulin sensitivity.
3. Poor Diet: Diets high in processed foods and added sugars can promote insulin resistance.
4. Chronic Stress: Stress hormones can interfere with insulin's action.
5. Genetics: Some genetic factors can predispose individuals to insulin resistance.

6.1.4 The Progression to Type 2 Diabetes

Insulin resistance doesn't immediately lead to diabetes. The progression typically follows these stages:

1. Normal blood sugar with increasing insulin resistance
2. Prediabetes (slightly elevated blood sugar)
3. Type 2 diabetes (significantly elevated blood sugar)

This progression can take years, providing opportunities for intervention and prevention.

6.2 Risk Factors and Warning Signs

Understanding the risk factors and recognizing early warning signs are crucial for preventing or managing type 2 diabetes effectively.

6.2.1 Risk Factors

Several factors can increase your risk of developing type 2 diabetes:

1. Age: Risk increases with age, especially after 45.
2. Family History: Having a close relative with type 2 diabetes increases your risk.
3. Ethnicity: Some ethnic groups have a higher risk, including African Americans, Hispanics, and Native Americans.
4. Obesity: Especially excess abdominal fat.
5. Sedentary Lifestyle: Lack of regular physical activity.
6. Diet: High consumption of processed foods, sugary drinks, and refined carbohydrates.
7. Gestational Diabetes: Women who had diabetes during pregnancy are at higher risk.
8. Polycystic Ovary Syndrome (PCOS): This hormonal disorder is associated with insulin resistance.
9. Sleep Disorders: Conditions like sleep apnea can increase risk.

6.2.2 Warning Signs

Early signs of type 2 diabetes can be subtle and easy to miss. They may include:

1. Increased Thirst: Your body tries to flush out excess glucose through urine, leading to dehydration and thirst.
2. Frequent Urination: Especially at night.
3. Increased Hunger: Despite eating, your cells may not be getting enough glucose.
4. Unexplained Weight Loss: When cells can't use glucose for energy, the body may break down muscle and fat.
5. Fatigue: Your cells aren't getting the energy they need from glucose.
6. Blurred Vision: High blood sugar can affect the shape of your eye's lens.
7. Slow-Healing Wounds: High blood sugar can impair the healing process.
8. Tingling or Numbness: In hands or feet, due to nerve damage from high blood sugar.
9. Darkened Skin Areas: Usually in the armpits and neck, a condition called acanthosis nigricans.

It's important to note that many people with type 2 diabetes may not experience any symptoms initially. Regular check-ups and blood tests are crucial for early detection.

6.3 The Long-term Consequences of Uncontrolled Diabetes

While type 2 diabetes can be managed effectively, uncontrolled diabetes can lead to serious long-term health complications affecting various parts of the body.

6.3.1 Cardiovascular Disease

People with diabetes are at higher risk of heart disease, stroke, and other cardiovascular problems. High blood sugar can damage blood vessels and the nerves that control the heart.

6.3.2 Kidney Disease (Nephropathy)

Diabetes can damage the kidneys' filtering system, potentially leading to kidney failure requiring dialysis or transplantation.

3.3.3 Eye Problems (Retinopathy and Cataracts)

High blood sugar can damage the blood vessels in the retina, potentially leading to vision loss. Diabetes also increases the risk of cataracts and glaucoma.

6.3.4 Nerve Damage (Neuropathy)

Excess sugar can injure the walls of tiny blood vessels that nourish nerves, especially in the legs. This can lead to tingling, numbness, burning or pain.

6.3.5 Foot Complications

Nerve damage and reduced blood flow can lead to serious foot problems, including increased risk of infections and, in severe cases, amputations.

6.3.6 Skin Conditions

Diabetes may make you more susceptible to skin problems, including bacterial and fungal infections.

6.3.7 Cognitive Decline

Research suggests that type 2 diabetes may increase the risk of dementia, including Alzheimer's disease.

6.3.8 Pregnancy Complications

For women, poorly controlled diabetes during pregnancy can lead to risks for both mother and baby.

6.3.9 The Importance of Management

These potential complications underscore the critical importance of proper diabetes management. With good blood sugar control, healthy lifestyle choices, and regular medical care, many of these complications can be delayed or prevented.

Understanding type 2 diabetes - its causes, risk factors, warning signs, and potential complications - is the first step toward effective prevention and management. In the following chapters, we'll explore strategies for maintaining metabolic health and, for those with diabetes, achieving better control and potentially even remission.

Chapter 7: The Current State of Diabetes Treatment

Diabetes mellitus, a chronic metabolic disorder characterized by elevated blood glucose levels, has become a global health crisis affecting millions of people worldwide. As our understanding of the disease has evolved, so too have the approaches to its treatment. This chapter explores the current landscape of diabetes management, examining standard medical approaches, their limitations, and the emerging concept of diabetes remission.

7.1 Standard Medical Approaches

The management of diabetes has traditionally focused on controlling blood glucose levels and preventing complications. The standard medical approaches vary depending on the type of diabetes and the individual patient's needs but generally include the following components:

7.1.1 Lifestyle Modifications

For all types of diabetes, lifestyle changes form the foundation of treatment. These include:
- Dietary adjustments: Emphasizing balanced nutrition, portion control, and carbohydrate management.
- Regular physical activity: Encouraging at least 150 minutes of moderate-intensity exercise per week.
- Weight management: Particularly important for individuals with type 2 diabetes or those at risk.

7.1.2 Blood Glucose Monitoring

- Regular monitoring of blood glucose levels is crucial for effective diabetes management. This may involve:
- Self-monitoring of blood glucose (SMBG) using glucometers.
- Continuous glucose monitoring (CGM) systems for real-time glucose tracking.
- Periodic HbA1c tests to assess long-term glucose control.

7.1.3 Pharmacological Interventions:

Medications play a vital role in managing diabetes, especially when lifestyle modifications alone are insufficient. Common pharmacological approaches include:

For Type 1 Diabetes
- Insulin therapy: Multiple daily injections or continuous subcutaneous insulin infusion (insulin pump therapy).

For Type 2 Diabetes
- Metformin: Often the first-line medication, improving insulin sensitivity.
- Sulfonylureas: Stimulating insulin production by the pancreas.
- DPP-4 inhibitors: Enhancing the body's ability to control blood sugar.
- GLP-1 receptor agonists: Slowing digestion and improving insulin production.
- SGLT2 inhibitors: Promoting glucose excretion through urine.

- Thiazolidinediones: Improving insulin sensitivity in body tissues.
- Insulin therapy: When other medications are inadequate.

7.1.4 Diabetes Education and Self-Management

Empowering patients with knowledge and skills to manage their condition effectively through:
- Diabetes self-management education and support (DSMES) programs.
- Nutritional counseling and meal planning guidance.
- Training in proper medication administration and glucose monitoring techniques.

7.1.5 Regular Medical Follow-ups

Ongoing medical supervision is essential for:
- Monitoring treatment efficacy and making necessary adjustments.
- Screening for and managing diabetes-related complications.
- Addressing comorbid conditions often associated with diabetes.

7.2 Limitations of Conventional Treatments

While the standard medical approaches have significantly improved the lives of many individuals with diabetes, they are not without limitations:

7.2.1 Glucose-Centric Focus

Conventional treatments primarily target blood glucose control, potentially overlooking other metabolic abnormalities associated with diabetes.

7.2.2 Progressive Nature of Type 2 Diabetes

Despite initial success with oral medications, many patients with type 2 diabetes eventually require insulin therapy as the disease progresses.

7.2.3 Side Effects and Complications

Some diabetes medications can cause undesirable side effects, such as weight gain, gastrointestinal issues, or hypoglycemia.

7.2.4 Treatment Burden

The complex regimen of multiple medications, frequent monitoring, and lifestyle adjustments can be overwhelming for patients, leading to poor adherence.

7.2.5 Cost and Accessibility

Advanced diabetes treatments and monitoring devices can be expensive and may not be accessible to all patients, particularly in resource-limited settings.

7.2.6 Incomplete Address of Underlying Causes

While conventional treatments manage symptoms effectively, they may not fully address the root causes of insulin resistance or beta-cell dysfunction in type 2 diabetes.

7.2.7 Psychological Impact

The chronic nature of diabetes management can lead to diabetes distress, affecting patients' mental health and quality of life.

7.2.8 Variability in Treatment Response

Individual responses to diabetes medications can vary significantly, necessitating a trial-and-error approach to find the optimal treatment regimen.

7.3 The Emerging Concept of Diabetes Remission

In recent years, a paradigm shift has occurred in diabetes management with the emergence of the concept of diabetes remission, particularly for type 2 diabetes. This approach aims not just to control the disease but to reverse its underlying pathophysiology.

7.3.1 Definition of Diabetes Remission

Diabetes remission is typically defined as achieving and maintaining normal blood glucose levels (HbA1c < 6.5%)

for at least three months without the use of glucose-lowering medications.

7.3.2 Approaches to Achieving Remission

Several strategies have shown promise in inducing diabetes remission:

a) Intensive Lifestyle Interventions:
-   Very low-calorie diets (VLCD) or low-carbohydrate diets.
-   Structured exercise programs.
-   Behavioral interventions for sustainable lifestyle changes.

b) Bariatric Surgery:
-   Procedures like Roux-en-Y gastric bypass and sleeve gastrectomy have demonstrated high rates of diabetes remission in obese individuals.

c) Pharmacological Approaches:
-   Early, aggressive treatment with combinations of medications targeting multiple pathways.
-   Novel therapies aimed at preserving or restoring beta-cell function.

7.3.3 Factors Influencing Remission

The likelihood of achieving remission appears to be influenced by:
-   Duration of diabetes: Earlier intervention tends to yield better results.
-   Degree of weight loss: Substantial weight reduction is often key to remission.

- Beta-cell function: Preserved insulin-producing capacity improves chances of remission.

7.3.4 Challenges and Considerations

While the concept of diabetes remission is promising, several challenges remain:
- Long-term sustainability of remission is uncertain and requires ongoing research.
- Not all individuals with type 2 diabetes may be able to achieve remission.
- The optimal approach to maintaining remission is still being explored.

7.3.5 Implications for Diabetes Care

The pursuit of diabetes remission is reshaping the landscape of diabetes management:
- Shifting focus from glucose control to addressing underlying pathophysiology.
- Emphasizing early, intensive interventions in newly diagnosed patients.
- Reconsidering treatment goals and success metrics in diabetes care.

As our understanding of diabetes continues to evolve, so too does our approach to its treatment. While conventional therapies remain the cornerstone of diabetes management for many, the emerging concept of diabetes remission offers hope for a future where diabetes may be not just managed, but potentially reversed. Ongoing research in this field promises to further refine our strategies and improve outcomes for individuals living with diabetes.

Part III: The Science Behind Metabolic Health

Chapter 8: Nutrition for Metabolic Health

Metabolic syndrome and type 2 diabetes are increasingly prevalent health concerns in modern society, largely driven by poor dietary habits, sedentary lifestyles, and genetic predisposition. This chapter explores the crucial role of nutrition in managing and potentially reversing these conditions, with a particular focus on dietary approaches such as low-carbohydrate, high-fat (LCHF) and carnivore diets.

8.1 The Role of Carbohydrates, Proteins, and Fats

8.1.1 Carbohydrates

Carbohydrates have long been a staple in human diets, but their overconsumption, particularly of refined and processed carbs, has been linked to the development of metabolic syndrome and type 2 diabetes. When consumed, carbohydrates are broken down into glucose, which enters the bloodstream and triggers an insulin response. In individuals with metabolic syndrome or type 2 diabetes, this insulin response can be impaired, leading to chronically elevated blood glucose levels.

The glycemic index (GI) and glycemic load (GL) are useful tools for understanding how different carbohydrates affect blood sugar levels. Low GI foods, such as non-starchy vegetables, legumes, and some fruits, cause a slower and more gradual rise in blood sugar compared to high GI foods like white bread, sugary snacks, and processed cereals.

In the context of metabolic health, many experts now advocate for significantly reducing carbohydrate intake, especially from refined sources. This approach forms the basis of low-carbohydrate diets, which have shown promise in improving insulin sensitivity, reducing inflammation, and promoting weight loss – all crucial factors in managing metabolic syndrome and type 2 diabetes.

8.1.2 Proteins

Proteins play a vital role in metabolic health. They are essential for building and repairing tissues, producing enzymes and hormones, and supporting immune function. Unlike carbohydrates, proteins have a minimal impact on blood sugar levels and can help promote feelings of fullness, potentially aiding in weight management.

In the context of metabolic syndrome and type 2 diabetes, adequate protein intake is crucial. It can help preserve muscle mass during weight loss, support stable blood sugar levels, and contribute to overall metabolic health. Sources of high-quality protein include lean meats, fish, eggs, dairy products, legumes, and some plant-based options like quinoa and soy.

Some studies suggest that higher protein diets may have benefits for individuals with metabolic syndrome or type 2 diabetes. These benefits include improved glycemic control, increased satiety, and better body composition. However, it's important to note that very high protein intakes may not be suitable for everyone, particularly those with kidney issues.

8.1.3 Fats

The role of dietary fat in metabolic health has been a subject of much debate and research in recent years. Contrary to past beliefs that advocated low-fat diets, current evidence suggests that certain types of fats can be beneficial for metabolic health, particularly when they replace refined carbohydrates in the diet.

Monounsaturated fats, found in foods like olive oil, avocados, and nuts, have been associated with improved insulin sensitivity and reduced inflammation. Omega-3 polyunsaturated fats, abundant in fatty fish, flaxseeds, and walnuts, have also shown benefits for metabolic health, including improved lipid profiles and reduced inflammation.

Even saturated fats, long vilified in nutritional guidelines, are being reevaluated. While excessive intake is still not recommended, moderate consumption of saturated fats from whole food sources (like grass-fed meat, coconut oil, and full-fat dairy) may not have the negative impacts once thought. Some studies have even suggested potential benefits, particularly when these fats replace refined carbohydrates in the diet.

The LCHF approach, which forms the basis of diets like the ketogenic diet, emphasizes high fat intake along with moderate protein and very low carbohydrate consumption. This dietary pattern aims to shift the body's primary fuel source from glucose to ketones, potentially offering benefits for blood sugar control, weight management, and overall metabolic health.

8.2 Micronutrients and Their Impact

While macronutrients often take center stage in discussions about metabolic health, micronutrients play equally crucial roles. Several vitamins and minerals are particularly important for individuals with metabolic syndrome or type 2 diabetes:

1. Magnesium: This mineral is involved in over 300 enzymatic reactions in the body, including those related to glucose metabolism and insulin sensitivity. Low magnesium levels have been associated with an increased risk of type 2 diabetes. Good sources include leafy greens, nuts, seeds, and whole grains.

2. Chromium: This trace mineral enhances the action of insulin and may improve glucose tolerance. It can be found in broccoli, grape juice, whole grains, and brewer's yeast.

3. Vitamin D: Often called the "sunshine vitamin," vitamin D plays a role in insulin sensitivity and secretion. Deficiency has been linked to an increased risk of metabolic syndrome and type 2 diabetes. While sunlight exposure is the primary source, it's also found in fatty fish, egg yolks, and fortified foods.

4. B-complex vitamins: These vitamins, particularly B1 (thiamine), B3 (niacin), and B12, are crucial for energy metabolism and may help improve insulin sensitivity. They are found in a variety of foods, including meat, eggs, leafy greens, and legumes.

5. Zinc: This mineral is involved in insulin synthesis, storage, and secretion. Good sources include oysters, beef, pumpkin seeds, and lentils.

6. Antioxidants: Vitamins C and E, along with other antioxidants like selenium and beta-carotene, help combat oxidative stress, which is often elevated in individuals with metabolic syndrome or type 2 diabetes. These can be found in a variety of fruits, vegetables, nuts, and seeds.

It's worth noting that while these micronutrients are important, they should ideally be obtained from whole food sources rather than supplements, unless otherwise recommended by a healthcare provider. A varied diet rich in nutrient-dense foods is typically the best approach to ensure adequate micronutrient intake.

8.3 Popular Diets: Keto, Low-Carb, Plant-Based, and More

Various dietary approaches have gained popularity for managing metabolic syndrome and type 2 diabetes. Here, we'll explore some of these diets, with a particular focus on low-carbohydrate, high-fat (LCHF) and carnivore diets:

8.3.1 Ketogenic Diet

The ketogenic diet is an extreme form of LCHF diet, typically consisting of about 70-80% of calories from fat, 15-20% from protein, and only 5-10% from carbohydrates. This severe carbohydrate restriction aims to induce a state of ketosis, where the body primarily burns fat for fuel instead of carbohydrates.

Potential benefits for metabolic health include:
- Improved insulin sensitivity
- Significant reductions in blood glucose levels
- Weight loss, particularly fat loss
- Reduced inflammation
- Improved lipid profiles (in many cases)

However, the ketogenic diet can be challenging to adhere to long-term and may not be suitable for everyone. It's important to implement this diet under medical supervision, especially for individuals with diabetes who may need to adjust their medications.

8.3.2 Low-Carb Diet

Less restrictive than the ketogenic diet, a general low-carb approach typically involves consuming less than 100-150g of carbohydrates per day. This can still offer many of the benefits of carbohydrate restriction without the potential challenges of maintaining ketosis.

- Benefits may include:
- Better blood sugar control
- Weight loss
- Improved insulin sensitivity
- Potential improvements in cardiovascular risk factors

8.3.3 Carnivore Diet:

The carnivore diet is an extreme form of low-carb eating that consists almost entirely of animal products. Proponents argue that it can lead to significant improvements in metabolic health, though it's important to note that long-term studies on this diet are limited.

Potential benefits claimed by advocates include:
- Rapid weight loss
- Improved insulin sensitivity
- Reduced inflammation
- Better mental clarity

However, the carnivore diet is highly restrictive and eliminates many nutrient-dense plant foods. It may pose risks of nutrient deficiencies and is not generally recommended by mainstream nutrition organizations.

8.3.4 Mediterranean Diet

While not specifically low-carb, the Mediterranean diet has shown benefits for metabolic health. It emphasizes:
- Olive oil as the primary fat source
- Abundant fruits, vegetables, and legumes
- Moderate amounts of fish and poultry
- Limited red meat
- Optional moderate red wine consumption

This diet has been associated with improved insulin sensitivity, better glycemic control, and reduced risk of cardiovascular disease.

8.3.5 Plant-Based Diets

Various plant-based diets, from vegetarian to vegan, have shown potential benefits for metabolic health. These diets typically:
- Are high in fiber, which can help with blood sugar control and satiety
- Are rich in antioxidants and phytonutrients, which may help reduce inflammation
- Often lead to weight loss, which can improve insulin sensitivity

However, poorly planned plant-based diets can be high in refined carbohydrates, which may negatively impact metabolic health. A well-planned, whole-food plant-based diet that's mindful of carbohydrate quality and quantity can be beneficial.

8.3.6 Intermittent Fasting

While not a specific diet, intermittent fasting has gained attention for its potential metabolic benefits. Various approaches exist, from time-restricted feeding to alternate-day fasting. Potential benefits include:
- Improved insulin sensitivity
- Weight loss
- Cellular repair processes (autophagy)

However, more research is needed on the long-term effects, and this approach may not be suitable for everyone, particularly those with a history of disordered eating.

8.4 Conclusion

When it comes to nutrition for metabolic health, there's no one-size-fits-all approach. While low-carbohydrate diets, including LCHF and carnivore diets, have shown promise for many individuals with metabolic syndrome or type 2 diabetes, other approaches can also be effective.

The key principles for most people include:
- Minimizing refined carbohydrates and added sugars
- Focusing on whole, nutrient-dense foods
- Ensuring adequate protein intake
- including healthy fats in the diet
- Paying attention to micronutrient intake

Ultimately, the best diet is one that's sustainable for the individual and leads to improved health markers. It's crucial to work with healthcare providers to find the right approach and monitor progress over time. Remember that diet is just one aspect of metabolic health – regular physical activity, stress management, and adequate sleep are also vital components of a comprehensive approach to managing metabolic syndrome and type 2 diabetes.

Physical activity is a cornerstone in the management and prevention of metabolic syndrome and type 2 diabetes. Regular exercise can dramatically improve metabolic health, insulin sensitivity, and overall quality of life for individuals facing these conditions. In this chapter, we'll explore the profound impact of exercise on metabolism, discuss different types of exercise, and guide you in creating an effective exercise routine.

Chapter 9: The Power of Physical Activity

9.1 How Exercise Affects Metabolism

Exercise has a multifaceted effect on metabolism, influencing both immediate and long-term metabolic processes. Understanding these effects can help motivate individuals to incorporate regular physical activity into their lives.

9.1.1 Immediate Effects

1. Increased Glucose Uptake: During exercise, muscles contract and require more energy. This leads to an immediate increase in glucose uptake from the bloodstream, even without insulin. This process, known as contraction-mediated glucose uptake, can help lower blood sugar levels during and shortly after exercise.

2. Enhanced Insulin Sensitivity: Exercise makes your body's cells more responsive to insulin. This means that less insulin is needed to move glucose from the bloodstream into cells, which is particularly beneficial for those with insulin resistance.

3. Elevated Metabolic Rate: Physical activity increases your metabolic rate, causing you to burn more calories during the activity and for several hours afterward. This phenomenon is known as excess post-exercise oxygen consumption (EPOC) or the "afterburn effect."

9.1.2 Long-term Effects

1. Improved Mitochondrial Function: Regular exercise increases the number and efficiency of

mitochondria, the cellular powerhouses responsible for energy production. This leads to better overall metabolic health and energy utilization.

2. Enhanced Fat Oxidation: Consistent exercise training improves your body's ability to use fat as fuel, which can help with weight management and reduce the risk of metabolic syndrome.

3. Increased Muscle Mass: Particularly with resistance training, exercise can lead to increased muscle mass. Muscle tissue is metabolically active, meaning it burns more calories even at rest, contributing to a higher basal metabolic rate.

4. Better Glycemic Control: Over time, regular exercise can lead to improved long-term blood sugar control, as measured by HbA1c levels in individuals with type 2 diabetes.

5. Reduced Inflammation: Chronic low-grade inflammation is often associated with metabolic syndrome and type 2 diabetes. Regular physical activity has anti-inflammatory effects, potentially reducing the risk of complications associated with these conditions.

6. Improved Cardiovascular Health: Exercise strengthens the heart and improves circulation, reducing the risk of cardiovascular complications often associated with metabolic syndrome and type 2 diabetes.

9.2 Types of Exercise: Aerobic vs. Resistance Training

Both aerobic exercise and resistance training play crucial roles in managing metabolic syndrome and type 2 diabetes. Each type of exercise offers unique benefits, and a combination of both is often recommended for optimal results.

9.2.1 Aerobic Exercise

Also known as cardio, aerobic exercise involves continuous, rhythmic movements that elevate your heart rate and breathing. Examples include walking, jogging, cycling, swimming, and dancing.

Benefits of Aerobic Exercise:
1. Improved Cardiovascular Health: Strengthens the heart and improves circulation.
2. Enhanced Insulin Sensitivity: Increases glucose uptake by muscles and improves insulin action.
3. Better Glycemic Control: Helps lower blood sugar levels during and after exercise.
4. Increased Calorie Burn: Aids in weight management and fat loss.
5. Reduced Blood Pressure: Helps lower both systolic and diastolic blood pressure.
6. Improved Cholesterol Profile: Can increase HDL (good) cholesterol and lower LDL (bad) cholesterol.

Recommended Aerobic Exercise:

- Aim for at least 150 minutes of moderate-intensity or 75 minutes of vigorous-intensity aerobic exercise per week.
- Spread activities throughout the week, with no more than two consecutive days without exercise.
- Start with shorter sessions (10-15 minutes) and gradually increase duration and intensity.

9.2.2 Resistance Training:

Also known as strength training, resistance training involves exercises that work muscles against a weight or force. This can include bodyweight exercises, free weights, resistance bands, or weight machines.

Benefits of Resistance Training:
1. Increased Muscle Mass: Builds and maintains lean muscle tissue.
2. Improved Insulin Sensitivity: Enhances glucose uptake and storage in muscles.
3. Higher Metabolic Rate: Increases basal metabolic rate due to increased muscle mass.
4. Better Body Composition: Helps reduce body fat percentage.
5. Enhanced Bone Density: Reduces the risk of osteoporosis, a concern for some individuals with diabetes.
6. Improved Functional Strength: Enhances ability to perform daily activities.

Recommended Resistance Training:
- Aim for at least two non-consecutive days of resistance training per week.
- Target all major muscle groups (legs, hips, back, abdomen, chest, shoulders, and arms).

- Start with lighter weights and focus on proper form before progressing.
- Aim for 2-3 sets of 8-12 repetitions for each exercise.

9.3 Finding the Right Exercise Routine

Creating an effective exercise routine for individuals with metabolic syndrome or type 2 diabetes requires careful consideration of their current fitness level, preferences, and any existing health concerns. Here are some guidelines to help develop an appropriate exercise plan:

1. Start Slowly: If you're new to exercise or have been inactive, start with low-intensity activities and gradually increase duration and intensity over time. This approach helps prevent injury and builds confidence.

2. Combine Aerobic and Resistance Training: Aim for a balanced program that includes both types of exercise. For example, you might do aerobic exercise 3-5 days a week and resistance training 2-3 days a week.

3. Monitor Blood Glucose: Check blood sugar levels before, during (for longer sessions), and after exercise, especially when starting a new routine. This helps you understand how different activities affect your glucose levels.

4. Stay Hydrated: Drink water before, during, and after exercise to prevent dehydration, which can affect blood glucose levels.

5. Time Your Exercise: For many people with type 2 diabetes, exercising 1-3 hours after a meal, when blood glucose tends to be elevated, can help with glucose control.

6. Listen to Your Body: Pay attention to how you feel during and after exercise. If you experience dizziness, unusual fatigue, or chest pain, stop exercising and consult your healthcare provider.

7. Choose Activities You Enjoy: You're more likely to stick with an exercise routine if you enjoy the activities. This might include group fitness classes, team sports, or outdoor activities like hiking.

8. Set Realistic Goals: Establish both short-term and long-term goals. These could be related to frequency of exercise, duration, intensity, or specific health markers like HbA1c levels.

9. Use Technology: Consider using fitness trackers or smartphone apps to monitor your activity levels and progress.

10. Seek Professional Guidance: Consult with a certified fitness professional who has experience working with individuals with metabolic syndrome or type 2 diabetes. They can help design a safe and effective program tailored to your needs.

11. Be Consistent: Regular, consistent exercise is key to seeing improvements in metabolic health. Aim to make physical activity a part of your daily routine.

12. Incorporate Daily Movement: Beyond structured exercise sessions, look for ways to increase your overall daily activity. This might include taking the stairs instead of the elevator, parking farther away from your destination, or doing active chores around the house.

Remember, the best exercise routine is one that you can stick to consistently. It's okay to start small and gradually build up your fitness level. The most important thing is to make regular physical activity a part of your lifestyle.

By understanding how exercise affects your metabolism, choosing the right types of activities, and finding an exercise routine that works for you, you can harness the power of physical activity to manage metabolic syndrome and type 2 diabetes effectively. Always consult with your healthcare provider before starting a new exercise program, especially if you have any complications related to your condition.

Chapter 10: Beyond Diet and Exercise

While diet and exercise are fundamental pillars in managing metabolic syndrome and type 2 diabetes, other factors play crucial roles in overall metabolic health. This chapter explores three key areas that can significantly impact your metabolism and overall well-being: sleep, stress management, and the gut microbiome.

10.1 The Impact of Sleep on Metabolism

Sleep is a vital yet often overlooked component of metabolic health. Adequate, quality sleep is essential for maintaining proper metabolic function and can significantly influence the management of metabolic syndrome and type 2 diabetes.

10.1.1 Sleep Duration and Metabolic Health

Research has consistently shown that both short and long sleep durations are associated with an increased risk of metabolic disorders. The optimal sleep duration for most adults is between 7-9 hours per night. Chronic sleep deprivation can lead to:

1. Insulin resistance: Lack of sleep can reduce insulin sensitivity, making it harder for your body to regulate blood glucose levels effectively.

2. Increased appetite: Sleep deprivation alters the production of hunger hormones, specifically increasing ghrelin (the "hunger hormone") and decreasing leptin (the "satiety hormone"). This can lead to overeating and weight gain.

3. Hormonal imbalances: Inadequate sleep can disrupt the balance of cortisol, growth hormone,

and thyroid-stimulating hormone, all of which play crucial roles in metabolism.

4. Inflammation: Chronic sleep deprivation can increase inflammatory markers in the body, which are associated with insulin resistance and cardiovascular risk.

10.1.2 Sleep Quality and Metabolic Function:

It's not just about how long you sleep, but also the quality of your sleep. Poor sleep quality, even if you're in bed for the recommended duration, can negatively impact metabolic health. Factors affecting sleep quality include:

1. Sleep apnea: This condition, characterized by repeated pauses in breathing during sleep, is common in individuals with obesity and type 2 diabetes. It can lead to fragmented sleep and is associated with insulin resistance and cardiovascular risk.

2. Circadian rhythm disruption: Irregular sleep schedules, shift work, and exposure to blue light at night can disrupt your body's natural circadian rhythm, affecting hormone production and metabolism.

3. Environmental factors: Noise, light, and temperature in your sleeping environment can all impact sleep quality and, consequently, metabolic function.

Improving Sleep for Better Metabolic Health:
To enhance your sleep and support your metabolic health:

1. Establish a consistent sleep schedule: Go to bed and wake up at the same time every day, even on weekends.

2. Create a sleep-friendly environment: Ensure your bedroom is dark, quiet, and cool.

3. Limit screen time before bed: The blue light emitted by electronic devices can interfere with melatonin production.

4. Avoid caffeine and large meals close to bedtime: These can disrupt your ability to fall asleep and the quality of your sleep.

5. Exercise regularly: Physical activity can improve sleep quality, but avoid vigorous exercise close to bedtime.

6. Manage stress: High stress levels can interfere with sleep, so incorporate stress-reduction techniques into your daily routine.

7. Consider sleep apnea screening: If you snore loudly or feel excessively tired during the day, consult your healthcare provider about sleep apnea testing.

10.2 Stress Management and Hormonal Balance

Chronic stress can have profound effects on metabolic health, particularly for those managing metabolic syndrome and type 2 diabetes. Understanding the relationship between stress and metabolism is crucial for developing effective management strategies.

10.2.1 The Stress-Metabolism Connection

When you experience stress, your body releases stress hormones like cortisol and adrenaline. While these hormones are essential for the "fight or flight" response, chronic elevation can lead to:

1. Insulin resistance: Cortisol can interfere with insulin's ability to regulate blood glucose, potentially exacerbating diabetes symptoms.

2. Increased appetite: Stress often leads to cravings for high-calorie, comfort foods, which can contribute to weight gain and poor glycemic control.

3. Visceral fat accumulation: Chronic stress is associated with increased deposition of fat around the abdominal organs, a key feature of metabolic syndrome.

4. Inflammation: Stress can promote systemic inflammation, which is linked to insulin resistance and cardiovascular risk.

5. Sleep disruption: High stress levels can interfere with sleep quality, creating a vicious cycle that further impacts metabolic health.

10.2.2 Hormonal Imbalances and Metabolism

Stress doesn't just affect cortisol; it can disrupt the delicate balance of various hormones that regulate metabolism:

1. Thyroid hormones: Chronic stress can suppress thyroid function, leading to a slower metabolism.

2. Growth hormone: Stress can interfere with the nighttime release of growth hormone, which plays a role in fat metabolism and muscle maintenance.

3. Sex hormones: Stress can affect the production of testosterone and estrogen, which influence body composition and insulin sensitivity.

10.2.3 Stress Management Strategies

Incorporating stress management techniques into your daily routine can significantly improve metabolic health:

1. Mindfulness and meditation: Regular practice can reduce stress hormones and improve insulin sensitivity.

2. Physical activity: Exercise is a powerful stress reducer and directly benefits metabolic health.

3. Deep breathing exercises: These can activate the parasympathetic nervous system, countering the stress response.

4. Progressive muscle relaxation: This technique can help reduce muscle tension and promote relaxation.

5. Social connections: Strong social support can buffer against the negative effects of stress.

6. Time in nature: Spending time outdoors has been shown to reduce stress hormones and improve overall well-being.

7. Cognitive Behavioral Therapy (CBT): This form of therapy can help you develop coping strategies for managing stress.

8. Adequate sleep: As discussed earlier, good sleep hygiene is crucial for stress management and metabolic health.

9. Hobbies and leisure activities: Engaging in enjoyable activities can reduce stress and improve overall quality of life.

10. Time management: Effective planning and prioritization can reduce daily stressors.

Implementing these strategies can help balance your stress hormones, potentially improving insulin sensitivity, reducing inflammation, and supporting overall metabolic health.

10.3 The Gut Microbiome and Metabolic Health

The gut microbiome, the vast community of microorganisms living in our digestive tract, plays a significant role in metabolic health. Recent research has revealed intricate connections between gut bacteria and various aspects of metabolism, including glucose regulation, appetite control, and inflammation.

10.3.1 The Gut-Metabolism Connection

Your gut microbiome influences metabolism through several mechanisms:

1. Short-chain fatty acid (SCFA) production: Certain gut bacteria ferment dietary fiber to produce SCFAs, which can improve insulin sensitivity and reduce inflammation.

2. Bile acid metabolism: The microbiome affects bile acid composition, which influences glucose and lipid metabolism.

3. Gut barrier function: A healthy microbiome maintains the integrity of the intestinal lining, preventing "leaky gut" and associated inflammation.

4. Appetite regulation: Gut bacteria can influence the production of hormones that control hunger and satiety.

5. Glucose metabolism: Some gut bacteria can directly affect blood glucose levels and insulin sensitivity.

10.3.2 Dysbiosis and Metabolic Disorders

Dysbiosis, an imbalance in the gut microbiome, has been associated with various metabolic disorders:

1. Obesity: Certain gut bacterial compositions are linked to increased risk of obesity.

2. Type 2 diabetes: Dysbiosis is common in individuals with diabetes and may contribute to insulin resistance.

3. Non-alcoholic fatty liver disease: Alterations in the gut microbiome are associated with this condition, which often coexists with metabolic syndrome.

4. Inflammation: An unhealthy gut microbiome can promote systemic inflammation, exacerbating metabolic issues.

10.3.3 Improving Gut Health for Metabolic Benefits

To support a healthy gut microbiome and potentially improve metabolic health:

1. Increase dietary fiber: Consume a variety of fruits, vegetables, whole grains, and legumes to provide prebiotics for beneficial bacteria.

2. Include fermented foods: Yogurt, kefir, sauerkraut, and kimchi can introduce beneficial bacteria to your gut.

3. Limit processed foods: Highly processed foods can negatively impact the gut microbiome.

4. Stay hydrated: Adequate water intake supports a healthy gut environment.

5. Consider probiotic supplements: Consult with your healthcare provider about whether probiotic supplementation might be beneficial for you.

6. Manage stress: Chronic stress can negatively impact the gut microbiome, so employ stress-reduction techniques.

7. Get regular exercise: Physical activity can promote a diverse and healthy gut microbiome.

8. Avoid unnecessary antibiotics: While sometimes necessary, antibiotics can disrupt the gut microbiome.

9. Practice good sleep hygiene: Quality sleep is associated with a healthier gut microbiome.

10. Explore prebiotic foods: Foods like garlic, onions, and leeks contain compounds that feed beneficial gut bacteria.

By focusing on these three areas – sleep, stress management, and gut health – in addition to diet and exercise, you can take a more comprehensive approach to managing metabolic syndrome and type 2 diabetes. Remember, these factors are interconnected, and improvements in one area often lead to benefits in others.

Chapter 11: Emerging Therapies and Research

The landscape of metabolic health is rapidly evolving, with new therapies and research continually emerging to address the growing concerns of metabolic syndrome and type 2 diabetes. This chapter explores some of the most promising approaches that are currently being investigated or implemented.

11.1 Intermittent Fasting and Time-Restricted Eating

Intermittent fasting (IF) and time-restricted eating (TRE) have gained significant attention in recent years as potential strategies for improving metabolic health. These approaches focus on when we eat rather than just what we eat, introducing periods of fasting into our daily or weekly routines.

11.1.1 Intermittent Fasting

IF involves alternating periods of eating and fasting. Several methods exist, including:

1. 16/8 method: Fasting for 16 hours and eating within an 8-hour window daily.
2. 5:2 diet: Eating normally for five days and restricting calories to 500-600 for two non-consecutive days per week.
3. Eat-Stop-Eat: Incorporating one or two 24-hour fasts per week.

Research has shown that IF can lead to improvements in insulin sensitivity, reduced inflammation, and weight loss. A study published in the New England Journal of Medicine in

2019 found that IF can trigger a metabolic switch from glucose-based to ketone-based energy, with associated improvements in health and aging processes.

11.1.2 Time-Restricted Eating

TRE involves limiting daily food intake to a specific window, typically 8-12 hours. This approach aligns eating patterns with circadian rhythms, potentially optimizing metabolic function.

A 2018 study in the journal Cell Metabolism demonstrated that TRE improved metabolic health in men with prediabetes, even without weight loss. Participants showed improved insulin sensitivity, blood pressure, and oxidative stress markers.

11.1.3 Mechanisms and Benefits

Both IF and TRE may improve metabolic health through several mechanisms:

1. Enhanced insulin sensitivity
2. Increased fat oxidation
3. Reduced inflammation
4. Improved circadian rhythm regulation
5. Autophagy stimulation (cellular "cleanup" process)

While promising, it's important to note that more long-term studies are needed to fully understand the effects of these approaches on metabolic health, especially in diverse populations.

11.2 Supplements and Nutraceuticals

As research progresses, certain supplements and nutraceuticals have shown potential in supporting metabolic health. Here are some noteworthy examples:

1. Berberine:

Berberine, a compound found in several plants, has gained attention for its potential to improve insulin sensitivity and glucose metabolism. A meta-analysis published in the Journal of Ethnopharmacology in 2015 found that berberine was as effective as metformin in improving glycemic control in type 2 diabetes patients.

2. Omega-3 Fatty Acids:

While not new, ongoing research continues to support the benefits of omega-3s for metabolic health. A 2021 study in Nature Communications found that omega-3 supplementation can help reduce liver fat and improve metabolic health markers in people with non-alcoholic fatty liver disease.

3. Resveratrol:

This polyphenol, found in red wine and grapes, has shown promise in improving insulin sensitivity and reducing inflammation. A 2019 meta-analysis in Nutrients suggested that resveratrol supplementation may improve glycemic control and cardiovascular risk factors in people with type 2 diabetes.

4. Curcumin:

The active compound in turmeric has demonstrated anti-inflammatory and antioxidant properties. A 2019 review in Foods highlighted curcumin's potential in managing metabolic syndrome through multiple pathways, including improved insulin sensitivity and reduced oxidative stress.

5. Probiotics and Prebiotics:
Emerging research is uncovering the crucial role of gut microbiota in metabolic health. A 2020 review in Nutrients discussed how specific probiotic strains and prebiotic fibers might help improve glycemic control and reduce inflammation in metabolic disorders.

While these supplements show promise, it's crucial to remember that they should not replace a healthy diet and lifestyle. More research is needed to establish optimal dosages and long-term effects, and individuals should consult healthcare providers before starting any new supplement regimen.

11.3 Promising Areas of Future Research

The field of metabolic health is dynamic, with several exciting areas of research that could lead to breakthrough therapies in the coming years:

1. Gut Microbiome Modulation:
The intricate relationship between gut microbiota and metabolic health is an area of intense research. Future therapies may involve personalized probiotics, prebiotics, or even fecal microbiota transplants to optimize metabolic function.

2. Epigenetic Interventions:

Researchers are exploring how environmental factors and lifestyle choices can influence gene expression related to metabolic health. This could lead to targeted interventions that "switch on" beneficial genes or "switch off" harmful ones.

3. Brown Fat Activation:
Brown adipose tissue, which burns calories to generate heat, is being studied for its potential in improving metabolic health. Future therapies might focus on increasing brown fat activity or converting white fat to brown fat.

4. Incretin Mimetics and GLP-1 Receptor Agonists:
While some GLP-1 receptor agonists are already in use for diabetes management, research is ongoing to develop more effective and longer-acting versions. These drugs show promise not only for glycemic control but also for weight management and cardiovascular health.

5. Senolytic Therapies:
The accumulation of senescent cells is associated with age-related metabolic decline. Senolytic drugs, which selectively eliminate these cells, are being studied for their potential to improve metabolic health and extend healthspan.

6. Nanotechnology:
Nanoparticles are being explored for targeted drug delivery and glucose monitoring. Future applications could include "smart" insulin delivery systems that respond in real-time to blood glucose levels.

7. Artificial Intelligence and Machine Learning:

These technologies are being applied to analyze large datasets, potentially leading to more personalized approaches to metabolic health management and early prediction of metabolic disorders.

8. Mitochondrial Therapeutics:
Given the central role of mitochondria in metabolism, researchers are exploring ways to enhance mitochondrial function. This could involve both pharmacological approaches and lifestyle interventions.

9. Circadian Rhythm Optimization:
Building on the concept of time-restricted eating, future therapies might involve more sophisticated ways to align various aspects of metabolism with circadian rhythms, potentially through light therapy, timed medication delivery, or chronotherapy.

10. CRISPR and Gene Therapy:
While still in early stages for metabolic disorders, gene editing technologies like CRISPR hold promise for correcting genetic factors contributing to metabolic syndrome and type 2 diabetes.

11.4 Conclusion

The field of metabolic health is at an exciting juncture, with emerging therapies and ongoing research offering new hope for individuals with metabolic syndrome and type 2 diabetes. From lifestyle interventions like intermittent fasting to cutting-edge areas like epigenetics and nanotechnology, the future holds the potential for more personalized, effective approaches to metabolic health management.

As research progresses, it's crucial for healthcare providers and patients to stay informed about these developments. However, it's equally important to remember that the foundations of good metabolic health – a balanced diet, regular physical activity, stress management, and adequate sleep – remain paramount. These emerging therapies and areas of research should be viewed as potential tools to complement, not replace, these fundamental lifestyle factors.

Chapter 12: Tracking Progress and Adjusting Course

For individuals managing metabolic syndrome and type 2 diabetes, monitoring progress and making necessary adjustments are crucial steps in the journey towards improved metabolic health. This chapter will explore the key metrics to track, when and how to adjust your approach, and the importance of medical supervision throughout this process.

12.1 Key Metrics to Monitor

Tracking specific health indicators is essential for understanding how your body responds to lifestyle changes and treatments. Here are the primary metrics you should monitor:

1. Blood Glucose Levels:
- Fasting blood glucose: Measure upon waking, before eating or drinking.
- Postprandial glucose: Check 1-2 hours after meals to assess how food affects your blood sugar.
- Hemoglobin A1C: This test provides an average of your blood glucose levels over the past 2-3 months.

2. Blood Pressure:
- Systolic and diastolic pressure: Monitor regularly, ideally at the same time each day.

3. Lipid Profile:
- Total cholesterol
- LDL (low-density lipoprotein) cholesterol
- HDL (high-density lipoprotein) cholesterol
- Triglycerides

4. Body Composition:

- Weight: Track consistently, preferably at the same time each day.
- Waist circumference: Measure at the level of your belly button.
- Body fat percentage: If possible, use methods like DEXA scans or bioelectrical impedance for accuracy.

5. Insulin Levels:
- Fasting insulin: This can help assess insulin sensitivity.
- HOMA-IR (Homeostatic Model Assessment of Insulin Resistance): Calculated using fasting glucose and insulin levels.

6. Liver Function:
- ALT (alanine aminotransferase) and AST (aspartate aminotransferase): These enzymes can indicate liver health.

7. Inflammatory Markers:
- High-sensitivity C-reactive protein (hs-CRP): An indicator of systemic inflammation.

8. 8. Nutritional Status:
- Vitamin D levels
- Magnesium levels
- Omega-3 index

9. Sleep Quality:
- Duration of sleep
- Sleep efficiency (time asleep vs. time in bed)
- Sleep stages (if using a sleep tracker)

10. Physical Activity:
- Steps per day
- Minutes of moderate to vigorous exercise
- Strength training sessions

11. Stress Levels:
- Subjective stress scores
- Heart rate variability (HRV) if available

By consistently tracking these metrics, you can gain valuable insights into your metabolic health progress and identify areas that may need more attention or adjustment.

12.2 When and How to Adjust Your Approach

Knowing when and how to adjust your approach is crucial for long-term success in managing metabolic syndrome and type 2 diabetes. Here are some guidelines:

1. Timing of Adjustments:
- Short-term fluctuations: Don't make drastic changes based on day-to-day variations. Look for trends over weeks or months.
- Plateaus: If you've been consistent with your approach but see no progress for 3-4 weeks, it may be time to adjust.
- Significant changes: If you notice sudden, unexplained changes in your metrics, consult your healthcare provider immediately.

2. Blood Glucose Management:
- If fasting glucose remains consistently above target: Consider adjusting medication timing,

evening meal composition, or discussing medication changes with your doctor.
- For postprandial spikes: Experiment with meal timing, composition, or pre-meal walks to improve glucose response.

3. Dietary Adjustments:
- Macronutrient ratios: If weight loss stalls or blood glucose control is suboptimal, consider adjusting your carbohydrate, protein, and fat intake.
- Meal timing: Experiment with meal frequency and timing to find what works best for your glucose control and energy levels.
- Food choices: Identify and eliminate foods that may be triggering inflammation or glucose spikes.

4. Exercise Modifications:
- Intensity: If you've plateaued, try increasing the intensity of your workouts.
- Variety: Incorporate different types of exercise to challenge your body in new ways.
- Timing: Experiment with exercise timing in relation to meals to optimize glucose control.

5. Sleep Optimization:
- If sleep quality is poor, focus on improving sleep hygiene, adjusting bedroom environment, or discussing potential sleep disorders with your doctor.

6. Stress Management:
- If stress levels remain high, consider incorporating additional stress-reduction techniques like meditation, yoga, or counseling.

7. Medication Adjustments:
-   Never adjust medications without consulting your healthcare provider.
-   If your metrics are consistently out of range despite lifestyle changes, discuss potential medication adjustments with your doctor.

8. Supplement Regimen:
-   Based on your nutritional status and overall health markers, work with your healthcare provider to adjust your supplement routine as needed.

Remember, adjustments should be made one at a time to clearly understand their impact. Give each change at least 2-4 weeks before assessing its effectiveness, unless you experience adverse effects that require immediate attention.

12.3 The Importance of Medical Supervision

While self-monitoring and making lifestyle adjustments are crucial for managing metabolic syndrome and type 2 diabetes, medical supervision remains an essential component of your health journey. Here's why:

1. Expertise and Guidance:
-   Healthcare providers have specialized knowledge to interpret complex health data and recommend evidence-based interventions.
-   They can help you set realistic goals and create personalized treatment plans.

2. Medication Management:
- Only licensed healthcare providers can prescribe and adjust medications.
- They can monitor for potential side effects and drug interactions.

3. Comprehensive Health Assessment:
- Regular check-ups allow for a holistic view of your health, beyond just metabolic markers.
- Healthcare providers can screen for related complications or comorbidities.

4. Access to Advanced Diagnostics:
- Certain tests, like DEXA scans or advanced lipid panels, require medical orders and interpretation.

5. Safety Monitoring:
- Medical supervision ensures that your approach to managing metabolic health is safe and appropriate for your individual circumstances.

6. Emotional Support:
- Healthcare providers can offer support and resources for the emotional aspects of managing chronic conditions.

7. Coordination of Care:
- If you need to see multiple specialists, your primary care provider can coordinate your overall care plan.

8. Education and Resources:
- Healthcare providers can offer up-to-date information on new treatments, research, and self-management techniques.

9. Insurance and Documentation:
- Regular medical visits ensure proper documentation for insurance purposes and can help you access necessary treatments or devices.

10. Emergency Preparedness:
- Your healthcare team can help you create plans for managing your condition during illnesses, travel, or other special circumstances.

To make the most of medical supervision:

- Schedule regular check-ups, typically every 3-6 months for stable patients, or more frequently if adjusting treatments.
- Prepare for appointments by bringing your self-monitoring data and a list of questions or concerns.
- Be honest about your lifestyle habits, challenges, and any symptoms you're experiencing.
- Follow through with recommended tests and referrals.
- Discuss any alternative treatments or supplements you're considering before starting them.

Remember, while you are the primary driver of your health, your healthcare team is an invaluable resource and partner in your journey to improved metabolic health. Regular medical supervision, combined with diligent self-monitoring and a proactive approach to lifestyle management, provides the best foundation for long-term success in managing metabolic syndrome and type 2 diabetes.

Chapter 13: Sustaining Long-Term Success

Improving metabolic health is a journey, not a destination. For individuals with metabolic syndrome and type 2 diabetes, maintaining progress over the long term is crucial for lasting health benefits. This chapter explores strategies for overcoming common challenges and building a foundation for sustained success.

13.1 Dealing with Plateaus and Setbacks

Plateaus and setbacks are normal parts of any health improvement journey. Understanding how to navigate these challenges is key to long-term success.

13.1.1 Recognizing Plateaus

A plateau occurs when progress seems to stall despite continued efforts. For those managing metabolic syndrome or type 2 diabetes, this might manifest as:
- Stable blood glucose levels after a period of improvement
- Weight loss slowing or stopping
- No further improvements in blood pressure or lipid profiles

13.1.2 Strategies for Overcoming Plateaus

1. Reassess Your Approach: Review your current diet, exercise routine, and medication regimen. Small adjustments can often jumpstart progress.

2. Increase Exercise Intensity or Duration: Gradually challenging your body with more intense or longer workouts can help break through fitness plateaus.

3. Fine-tune Your Diet: Consider adjusting your macronutrient balance or meal timing. For example, experimenting with intermittent fasting or reducing carbohydrate intake might help improve insulin sensitivity.

4. Focus on Non-Scale Victories: Look for improvements in energy levels, sleep quality, or clothing fit. These can be motivating when weight loss slows.

5. Consult Your Healthcare Team: Regular check-ins with your doctor or dietitian can help identify any necessary adjustments to your treatment plan.

13.1.3 Handling Setbacks

Setbacks are temporary reversals in progress. They might include weight gain, elevated blood sugar levels, or a return of symptoms. When facing a setback:

1. Practice Self-Compassion: Avoid self-criticism. Remember that setbacks are a normal part of the process.

2. Identify Triggers: Analyze what led to the setback. Was it stress, a change in routine, or a specific event?

3. Return to Basics: Revisit the fundamental habits that initially led to improvements in your metabolic health.

4. Learn and Adapt: Use setbacks as learning opportunities to strengthen your long-term strategy.

5. Seek Support: Reach out to your healthcare team or support network for guidance and encouragement.

13.2 Building a Supportive Environment

Creating an environment that supports your health goals is crucial for long-term success in managing metabolic syndrome and type 2 diabetes.

13.2.1 Home Environment

1. Pantry Makeover: Stock your kitchen with healthy, whole foods. Remove or limit access to processed foods high in sugar and unhealthy fats.

2. Meal Prep Area: Designate a space for easy meal preparation, making it more convenient to cook healthy meals at home.

3. Exercise Space: Create a dedicated area for physical activity, even if it's just enough room for a yoga mat or some resistance bands.

4. Sleep Sanctuary: Optimize your bedroom for quality sleep, which is crucial for metabolic health.

13.2.2 Social Environment

1. Communicate Your Goals: Share your health objectives with friends and family, explaining why they're important to you.

2. Find Health-Minded Friends: Connect with others who share similar health goals, either in-person or through online communities.

3. Plan Social Activities Around Health: Suggest active outings or healthy cooking sessions when socializing.

4. Set Boundaries: Learn to politely decline offers that don't align with your health goals.

13.2.3 Workplace Environment

1. Healthy Snack Stash: Keep nutritious snacks at your desk to avoid unhealthy vending machine options.

2. Movement Breaks: Set reminders to stand up and move regularly throughout the workday.

3. Stress Management: Implement stress-reduction techniques like deep breathing or short meditation sessions during breaks.

4. Communicate with Colleagues: Let coworkers know about your health goals to minimize pressure to participate in unhealthy office habits.

13.3 The Psychological Aspects of Lifestyle Change

Sustainable lifestyle changes require not just physical adjustments, but also psychological adaptation. Understanding and managing the mental aspects of change is crucial for long-term success in improving metabolic health.

13.3.1 Mindset Shift

1. From Diet to Lifestyle: View your changes not as a temporary "diet" but as a permanent lifestyle improvement.
2. Progress, Not Perfection: Embrace small, consistent improvements rather than aiming for flawless adherence.
3. Identity Change: Begin to see yourself as a person who prioritizes health, rather than someone trying to become healthy.

13.3.2 Motivation Maintenance

1. Set Process Goals: Focus on actionable behaviors (e.g., "eat vegetables with every meal") rather than just outcome goals (e.g., "lose 20 pounds").

2. Celebrate Small Wins: Acknowledge and reward yourself for achieving milestones, no matter how small.
3. Visualize Success: Regularly imagine yourself achieving your health goals and enjoying the benefits.
4. Find Your 'Why': Connect your health goals to deeper personal values or life aspirations.

13.3.3 Emotional Management

1. Stress Reduction Techniques: Practice stress management methods like meditation, deep breathing, or progressive muscle relaxation.
2. Emotional Eating Awareness: Learn to recognize and address emotional triggers for unhealthy eating.
3. Cognitive Restructuring: Challenge and reframe negative thoughts about your health journey.
4. Mindfulness Practice: Develop mindfulness to stay present and make conscious choices about food and activity.

13.3.4 Building Habits

1. Start Small: Begin with tiny, manageable changes that can be easily integrated into your routine.
2. Use Habit Stacking: Attach new healthy habits to existing routines for easier adoption.
3. Create Environmental Cues: Use visual reminders or alarms to prompt desired behaviors.
4. Practice Consistency: Focus on performing health-promoting actions consistently, even if imperfectly.

13.3.5 Dealing with Social Pressure

1. Assertiveness Training: Learn to confidently communicate your needs and boundaries in social situations.
2. Prepare Responses: Have ready answers for common questions or pressures about your lifestyle choices.

3. Find Like-Minded Communities: Engage with support groups or online forums for individuals managing metabolic health.
4. Educate Others: Share information about metabolic health with friends and family to increase understanding and support.

13.3.6 Seeking Professional Support

1. Regular Check-ins: Schedule periodic visits with a therapist or counselor to address ongoing psychological challenges.

2. Cognitive Behavioral Therapy (CBT): Consider CBT to develop coping strategies and change negative thought patterns.
3. Health Coaching: Work with a health coach to set and achieve personalized health goals.
4. Support Groups: Participate in group therapy or support groups for individuals with metabolic syndrome or type 2 diabetes.

13.4 Conclusion

Sustaining long-term success in managing metabolic syndrome and type 2 diabetes requires a multifaceted approach. By effectively dealing with plateaus and setbacks, creating a supportive environment, and addressing the psychological aspects of lifestyle change, individuals can build a robust foundation for lasting health improvements. Remember that the journey to better metabolic health is ongoing, and each day presents a new opportunity to make choices that support your well-being. With patience, persistence, and the right strategies, long-term success in managing metabolic health is achievable.

A New Lease on Life

Reversing metabolic syndrome and type 2 diabetes through lifestyle changes has given me a new lease on life, a chance to live more fully and with greater awareness of my health. My journey has been one of discovery, discipline, and transformation. It has not only restored my physical health but also enriched my mental and emotional well-being.

Embracing Change

The initial diagnosis was a wake-up call—a stark reminder that our health is intricately linked to our lifestyle choices. Instead of succumbing to the despair of a lifelong dependency on medication, I chose to embrace change. I started by educating myself about the fundamental role that diet, exercise, sleep, and stress management play in managing and reversing metabolic syndrome and type 2 diabetes.

By eliminating processed foods, reducing sugar intake, and incorporating whole, nutrient-dense foods into my diet, I experienced significant improvements in my blood sugar levels and overall energy. Regular physical activity, tailored to my fitness level, helped in weight management and boosted my cardiovascular health. Prioritizing quality sleep and implementing stress reduction techniques, such as mindfulness and meditation, further complemented my efforts.

The Power of Self-Determination

This journey has underscored the power of self-determination and the human spirit's resilience. Each step, whether it was a dietary change or a new exercise routine, reinforced my belief that we possess the inherent ability to heal and thrive. The sense of control over my health outcomes empowered me, transforming fear and uncertainty into confidence and purpose.

My success was not an overnight miracle but the result of consistent, small changes. Celebrating each milestone, no matter how minor, kept me motivated. Over time, these small victories accumulated, leading to significant health improvements. This process taught me the value of patience and perseverance.

Advocating for Change

My transformation ignited a passion to help others. Realizing that my story could inspire and guide those facing similar challenges, I became an advocate for metabolic health. Through workshops, community meetings, and social media platforms, I shared my journey, emphasizing that lifestyle changes can lead to profound health benefits.

Advocacy is about more than sharing success stories; it is about fostering a supportive community. By listening to others' experiences and providing practical advice, I aimed to create an environment where individuals felt understood and motivated to embark on their own health journeys. Witnessing others' successes fueled my commitment to this cause.

The Broader Impact

Changing individual lives is rewarding, but the broader impact lies in shifting the collective mindset towards diabetes management. Advocacy efforts aim to change how healthcare providers, policymakers, and society at large view and address metabolic health. Encouraging a holistic approach that includes lifestyle changes alongside medical interventions can lead to more sustainable health outcomes.

A critical part of this paradigm shift is addressing the socio-economic factors that influence health. Advocacy must also focus on ensuring access to healthy foods, safe exercise environments, and affordable healthcare. This comprehensive approach is essential for creating an equitable and supportive framework for all individuals.

Looking Forward

As I reflect on my journey, I am filled with gratitude and hope. Gratitude for the knowledge, support, and resources that enabled my transformation, and hope for a future where more individuals can reclaim their health through informed and proactive choices.

My story is a testament to the fact that metabolic syndrome and type 2 diabetes do not have to be lifelong sentences. With the right mindset, resources, and support, these conditions can be managed and even reversed. My mission is to continue advocating for metabolic health, sharing knowledge, and supporting others on their paths to wellness.

In conclusion, my journey from diagnosis to health advocate has given me a profound sense of purpose. By embracing lifestyle changes and taking control of my health, I have experienced a new lease on life. My hope is that others will be inspired to embark on their own journeys, realizing that with determination and support, they too can achieve lasting health and well-being. Together, we can shift the paradigm and create a future where metabolic syndrome and type 2 diabetes are managed not just by drugs, but by empowered, informed lifestyle choices.

Additional Resources

Healthy recipes that I love !

1. Grilled Lemon Herb Chicken

Ingredients
- 4 boneless, skinless chicken breasts
- 2 tbsp olive oil
- 2 tbsp lemon juice
- 2 cloves garlic, minced
- 1 tsp dried oregano
- Salt and pepper to taste

Instructions
1. In a bowl, mix olive oil, lemon juice, garlic, oregano, salt, and pepper.
2. Marinate chicken breasts in the mixture for at least 30 minutes.
3. Grill the chicken over medium heat for 6-7 minutes on each side or until cooked through.

2. Quinoa and Black Bean Salad

Ingredients
- 1 cup quinoa, cooked
- 1 can black beans, drained and rinsed
- 1 cup cherry tomatoes, halved
- 1 bell pepper, diced
- 1 small red onion, diced
- 1 avocado, diced
- 2 tbsp olive oil
- 2 tbsp lime juice
- Salt and pepper to taste

Instructions
1. In a large bowl, combine quinoa, black beans, tomatoes, bell pepper, red onion, and avocado.
2. Drizzle with olive oil and lime juice, then season with salt and pepper. Toss to combine.

3. Baked Salmon with Asparagus

Ingredients
- 4 salmon fillets
- 1 bunch asparagus, trimmed
- 2 tbsp olive oil
- 2 cloves garlic, minced
- Salt and pepper to taste
- Lemon slices for garnish

Instructions
1. Preheat the oven to 400°F (200°C).
2. Place salmon fillets and asparagus on a baking sheet.
3. Drizzle with olive oil and sprinkle with garlic, salt, and pepper.
4. Bake for 15-20 minutes or until salmon is cooked through. Garnish with lemon slices.

4. Chickpea and Spinach Curry

Ingredients
- 1 can chickpeas, drained and rinsed
- 1 bag fresh spinach
- 1 can diced tomatoes
- 1 onion, chopped
- 2 cloves garlic, minced
- 1 tbsp curry powder
- 1 tsp ground cumin
- 1 tsp ground coriander
- Salt and pepper to taste

Instructions
1. In a large pan, sauté the onion and garlic until soft.
2. Add curry powder, cumin, and coriander, and cook for 1 minute.
3. Add chickpeas, tomatoes, and spinach. Simmer for 15 minutes.
4. Season with salt and pepper to taste.

5. Greek Yogurt and Berry Parfait

Ingredients
- 1 cup Greek yogurt
- 1/2 cup mixed berries (strawberries, blueberries, raspberries)
- 1 tbsp chia seeds
- 1 tbsp honey (optional)

Instructions
1. Layer Greek yogurt, mixed berries, and chia seeds in a glass or bowl.
2. Drizzle with honey if desired.

6. Turkey and Vegetable Stir-Fry

Ingredients
- 1 lb ground turkey
- 2 cups mixed vegetables (bell peppers, broccoli, carrots)
- 2 cloves garlic, minced
- 1 tbsp soy sauce (low sodium)
- 1 tbsp olive oil
- Salt and pepper to taste

Instructions
1. In a large pan, heat olive oil and cook garlic until fragrant.
2. Add ground turkey and cook until browned.
3. Add mixed vegetables and soy sauce. Stir-fry until vegetables are tender.
4. Season with salt and pepper to taste.

7. Cauliflower Rice Tabbouleh

Ingredients

- 1 head cauliflower, riced
- 1 cup chopped parsley
- 1/2 cup chopped mint
- 1/2 cup diced cucumber
- 1/2 cup diced tomatoes
- 2 tbsp olive oil
- 2 tbsp lemon juice
- Salt and pepper to taste

Instructions

1. In a large bowl, combine riced cauliflower, parsley, mint, cucumber, and tomatoes.
2. Drizzle with olive oil and lemon juice, then season with salt and pepper. Toss to combine.

8. Stuffed Bell Peppers

Ingredients
- 4 bell peppers, tops cut off and seeds removed
- 1 lb ground chicken
- 1 cup cooked quinoa
- 1 can diced tomatoes
- 1 onion, chopped
- 2 cloves garlic, minced
- 1 tsp paprika
- Salt and pepper to taste

Instructions
1. Preheat the oven to 375°F (190°C).
2. In a pan, cook the onion and garlic until soft.
3. Add ground chicken and cook until browned.
4. Stir in quinoa, diced tomatoes, paprika, salt, and pepper.
5. Stuff bell peppers with the mixture and place them in a baking dish.
6. Bake for 30-35 minutes.

9. Lentil Soup

Ingredients
- 1 cup lentils, rinsed
- 1 onion, chopped
- 2 carrots, diced
- 2 celery stalks, diced
- 2 cloves garlic, minced
- 1 can diced tomatoes
- 4 cups vegetable broth
- 1 tsp cumin
- 1 tsp thyme
- Salt and pepper to taste

Instructions
1. In a large pot, sauté onion, carrots, celery, and garlic until soft.
2. Add lentils, diced tomatoes, vegetable broth, cumin, and thyme.
3. Bring to a boil, then reduce heat and simmer for 30-40 minutes.
4. Season with salt and pepper to taste.

10. Zucchini Noodles with Pesto

Ingredients
- 4 zucchinis, spiralized
- 1 cup fresh basil
- 1/4 cup pine nuts
- 1/4 cup grated Parmesan cheese
- 2 cloves garlic
- 1/4 cup olive oil
- Salt and pepper to taste

Instructions
1. In a food processor, blend basil, pine nuts, Parmesan cheese, garlic, and olive oil until smooth.
2. In a pan, sauté zucchini noodles for 2-3 minutes.
3. Toss with pesto sauce and season with salt and pepper to taste.

Exercises for beginners

Cardio-respiratory training

1. Walking: A great starting point, especially for beginners. Try to maintain a brisk pace.
2. Jogging: Gradually increase your pace from walking to jogging to improve cardiovascular endurance.
3. Cycling: Whether on a stationary bike or outdoors, cycling is a low-impact exercise that can be adjusted for different fitness levels.
4. Swimming: Offers a full-body workout and is gentle on the joints. Aim for continuous laps with short breaks.
5. Jump Rope: An excellent way to get your heart rate up. Start with shorter intervals and gradually increase the duration.
6. Elliptical Training: Provides a low-impact workout that can be adjusted for intensity.
7. Rowing: Works the entire body and can be done on a rowing machine. Adjust resistance for different levels
8. Dancing: Follow along with dance workout videos or join a dance class for a fun and effective cardio workout.
9. Hiking: Great for building endurance and enjoying the outdoors. Choose trails that match your fitness level.
10. High-Intensity Interval Training (HIIT): Alternate between short bursts of intense activity and rest. Exercises like jumping jacks, burpees, and high knees can be included.

Remember to start at your own pace, gradually increase
the intensity, and always listen to your body to avoid injury.

Muscle and Strength training

1. Bodyweight Squats: Great for building leg strength. Start with bodyweight and progress to using weights.
2. Push-Ups: Effective for chest, shoulders, and triceps. Modify by starting on knees if needed.
3. Dumbbell Rows: Targets the back and biceps. Use a bench or any sturdy surface for support.
4. Lunges: Excellent for leg and glute strength. Start with bodyweight and progress to holding dumbbells.
5. Plank: Builds core strength. Begin with shorter durations and gradually increase the time.
6. Dumbbell Bench Press: Targets the chest, shoulders, and triceps. Use a bench and appropriate weights.
7. Bicep Curls: Focus on the biceps using dumbbells. Start with light weights and increase as you get stronger.
8. Tricep Dips: Great for triceps. Use a bench or sturdy chair for support.
9. Deadlifts: Effective for the entire posterior chain. Start with light weights and ensure proper form.
10. Shoulder Press: Strengthens the shoulders and triceps. Can be done with dumbbells or a barbell.

As with any strength training program, focus on proper form, start with lighter weights, and gradually increase the resistance as you become more comfortable and stronger.

Mobility and Flexibility training

1. Cat-Cow Stretch Great for spinal mobility and flexibility. Move between arching and rounding your back.
2. Hip Circles: Improves hip mobility. Stand or get on all fours and make circular movements with your hips.
3. Seated Forward Bend: Stretches the hamstrings and lower back. Sit with legs extended and reach for your toes.
4. Thoracic Spine Rotation: Enhances upper back mobility. Sit or lie on your side and rotate your upper body.
5. Child's Pose: A gentle stretch for the back, hips, and shoulders. Kneel and sit back on your heels while reaching forward.
6. Downward-Facing Dog: Stretches the hamstrings, calves, and shoulders. Form an inverted V shape with your body.
7. Hip Flexor Stretch: Stretches the hip flexors and improves hip mobility. Lunge forward and gently press your hips down.
8. Butterfly Stretch: Targets the inner thighs and groin. Sit with the soles of your feet together and gently press your knees down.
9. Triceps Stretch: Increases flexibility in the triceps and shoulders. Reach one arm overhead and bend the elbow, using the other hand to press the arm further.
10. Neck Stretches: Improves neck mobility and flexibility. Gently tilt your head from side to side and forward and backward.

Incorporate these exercises into your routine, aiming to hold each stretch for 20-30 seconds and repeating 2-3 times for each side or movement. Remember to breathe deeply and never force any stretch to the point of pain.

Recommended Resources

Books

1. [Metabolical: The Lure and the Lies of Processed Food, Nutrition, and Modern Medicine](#)
2. [Stay off My Operating Table: A Heart Surgeon's Metabolic Health Guide](#)
3. [UNHOLY TRINITY: How Carbs, Sugar & Oils Make Us Fat, Sick & Addicted and How to Escape Their Grip](#)
4. [Lies My Doctor Told Me Second Edition: Why We Get Fat: And What to Do About It by Gary Taubes](#)
5. [Outlive: The Science and Art of Longevity](#)

Websites

1. NutritionFacts.org
2. American Diabetes Association
3. Centers for Disease Control and Prevention (CDC) - Diabetes
4. Levels Health
5. Diet Doctor

Online Courses

1. <u>Coursera - "Diabetes – a Global Challenge" by University of Copenhagen</u>
2. <u>Udemy - "Nutrition Masterclass: Build Your Perfect Diet & Meal Plan</u>
3. <u>FutureLearn - "The Role of Diet and Nutrition in Type 2 Diabetes</u>

Podcasts

1. The Peter Attia Drive Podcast
2. The Doctor's Farmacy with Dr. Mark
3. FoundMyFitness with Dr. Rhonda Patrick
4. The Ultimate Health Podcast - Jesse Chappus
5. Huberman Lab Podcast

YouTube Channels

1. Dr. Ford Brewer
2. KenDBerryMD
3. Dr. Robert Cywes the #CarbAddictionDoc
4. Insulin IQ
5. Dr. Eric Berg DC
6. Peter Attia MD

Legal Disclaimer

The information provided in this book, titled **[*System Upgrade: Reprogramming Metabolism After 50*]**, is based on the author's personal experiences and research regarding metabolic health. The content is intended for informational and educational purposes only and should not be considered medical advice.

No Medical Advice

The author is not a licensed healthcare professional, and the information presented in this book is not a substitute for professional medical advice, diagnosis, or treatment. Readers are encouraged to consult with a qualified healthcare provider before making any changes to their diet, exercise, or health regimen.

Personal Journey

This book reflects the author's personal journey and experiences with metabolic health. Individual results may vary, and what works for one person may not work for another. The author does not guarantee specific outcomes or results from the information shared in this book.

Limitation of Liability

By reading this book, you acknowledge and agree that the author, publisher, and any affiliated parties are not liable for any adverse effects or consequences resulting from the use or application of any information presented herein. You assume full responsibility for your health and well-being and agree to seek professional guidance as necessary.

No Endorsements

Any references to products, services, or organizations in this book are for informational purposes only and do not constitute endorsements or recommendations by the author. The author does not receive compensation for any products mentioned.

Conclusion

Your health is your responsibility. Always seek the advice of your healthcare provider with any questions you may have regarding a medical condition or treatment.